MRCP PART 1 PAST TOPICS

A REVISION SYLLABUS

Second Edition

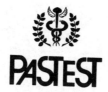

PASTEST

MRCP PART 1 PAST TOPICS
A REVISION SYLLABUS
Second Edition

Compiled and edited by

Philip A Kalra MA MB BChir MRCP MD
Consultant Nephrologist
Hope Hospital, The University of Manchester, Salford

First Edition 1996
Second Edition 1998

ISBN 1 901198 11 1

A catalogue record for this book is available from the British Library.

PasTest Revision Books and Intensive Courses

PasTest has been established in the field of postgraduate medical education since 1972, providing revision books and intensive study courses for doctors preparing for their professional examinations.
Books and courses are available for the following specialties:
MRCP Part 1 and Part 2 (General Medicine and Paediatrics), MRCOG, DRCOG, MRCGP, DCH, FRCA, MRCS, PLAB.
For further details contact:
**PasTest, Freepost, Knutsford, Cheshire WA16 7BR
Tel: 01565 755226   Fax: 01565 650264**

Text prepared by Breeze Limited, Manchester.
Printed by Athenaeum Press, Gateshead, Tyne and Wear

CONTENTS

A breakdown of the relative distribution of topics is given below. A slight variation may occur from exam to exam.

Subject Area	Number of MCQs
Neurology	5/6
Pharmacology	4/5
Cardiology	4/5
Basic Sciences	3/6
Gastroenterology	4/5
Respiratory Medicine	4
Infectious Diseases	4
Endocrinology	4
Psychiatry	3/4
Haematology	4
Nephrology	3/4
Metabolism	2/3
Immunology	2/3
Rheumatology	2
Genetics	1/2
Statistics	1
Dermatology	0/1
Ophthalmology	0/1
Total Number of MCQs	**60**

INTRODUCTION

The pass rate for candidates sitting the MRCP (UK) Part 1 examination is fixed, such that the top 35% are successful. As there are increasing numbers of entrants for each exam this encourages candidates to develop a highly competitive approach. Furthermore, the style of preparation for the examination is changing with a greater proportion of candidates attending courses that improve MCQ answering technique and question exposure; innumerable books of 'typical' MRCP MCQs are also available, and candidates can be swamped with 'likely topics' for forthcoming exams.

This book is markedly different from all previous Part 1 books, and provides a major advantage to candidates by indicating the topics most frequently used in past Royal College examinations. The material has been accumulated by amalgamating the feedback of candidates who have taken the exam after attending PasTest courses during the last seven years (1991–1997).

Exam topics are listed chronologically within each parent subject. These lists enable candidates to appreciate the spectrum of questions used in any one MRCP examination, and provide insight into topics which may be declining in popularity whilst others may be increasingly utilised (eg. inflammatory/vasoactive mediators), reflecting advances in medical science.

The second section within each chapter is a compilation of related topics under subheadings which will provide a comprehensive checklist for candidates that should enhance revision strategy – e.g. within *Nephrology* it would be sensible to concentrate more revision time on the nephrotic syndrome and related membranous/ minimal change glomerulonephritis (17 questions during last 7 years) than on renal bone disease (1 question during same period). Equally, it should become clear to candidates that prolonged revision of subjects such as *Ophthalmology* and *Dermatology* (only 1 question for either subject every 2 or 3 exams) will be less fruitful than concentrating on deficiencies in their knowledge of *Cardiology* and *Neurology* (10-11 questions in any exam).

There are inevitable overlaps, for example pulmonary manifestations of SLE or rheumatoid arthritis could appear in either of 2 sections; certain topics are cross-referenced. Many 'basic science' topics are also considered within the parent subject, such as renal tubular and respiratory physiology, and the effects of lesions involving/anatomy of cranial and peripheral nerves.

As there is no published syllabus available for this exam I hope that all MRCP Part 1 candidates will benefit from the focused revision that this book will facilitate.

P A Kalra

October 1997
    Prostacyclin
    Atrial natriuretic peptide
    Angiotensin and receptors

July 1997
    Organelles with self-replicating DNA

Jan 1997
    Apoptosis

October 1996
    Nitric oxide
    Neurotransmitters

July 1996
    Changes in pregnancy
    Nitric oxide

February 1996
    Aldosterone secretion

October 1995
    Physiology of late pregnancy

July 1995
    Steroid hormone receptors
    H_2 receptors
    Atrial natriuretic peptide

February 1995
    Amyloid plaques
    Apolipoprotein
    $Alpha_1$-antitrypsin

October 1994
The polymerase chain reaction
Actions of insulin
Endothelium derived relaxing factor (Nitric oxide)
Mitochondrial DNA
The RAS oncogene
Adenosine

February 1994
Somatostatin

October 1993
Oxygen uptake by haemoglobin
Physiology of normal bone
Atrial natriuretic peptide
Actions of insulin

July 1993
Serum ferritin
Angiotensin-II

February 1993
Function of hypothalamic nucleii

February 1992
Neurotransmitters
Physiological changes in normal pregnancy
Prostacyclin

October 1991
Peripheral oedema
Actions of ADH

February 1991
Atrial natriuretic peptide
Insulin resistance

Average 3-6 questions per exam (many questions involving anatomy/physiology of a specific topic included within that section). Numbers in brackets indicate the relative frequency of topics.

Physiology
- [ ] Changes in pregnancy (3)
- [ ] Haemoglobin function
- [ ] Physiology of bone
- [ ] Aetiology of oedema

Pathology
- [ ] Amyloid plaques
- [ ] Apoptosis

Hormone and mediator biochemistry
- [ ] Atrial natriuretic peptides (4)
- [ ] Insulin/insulin resistance (3)
- [ ] Nitric oxide (3)
- [ ] Angiotensin (2)
- [ ] Neurotransmitters (2)
- [ ] Prostacyclin (2)
- [ ] Adenosine
- [ ] ADH
- [ ] Aldosterone
- [ ] H2 receptors
- [ ] Somatostatin
- [ ] Steroid receptors

Miscellaneous
- [ ] Organelles with DNA (2)
- [ ] Apolipoproteins
- [ ] Alpha$_1$-antitrypsin
- [ ] Oncogenes

October 1997
   Causes of myocardial infarction
   Paroxysmal SVT
   Indicators of underlying heart disease
   Ischaemic heart disease
   Structure and physiology of carotid body

July 1997
   HOCM
   Cardiac tamponade
   Left atrial myxoma

Jan 1997
   Ostium secundum ASD
   Post-CABG
   Sympathetic cardiac stimulation
   Post-MI/cholesterol
   Atrial fibrillation
   LVH

October 1996
   Constrictive pericarditis
   Cardiac murmurs
   Primary pulmonary hypertension

July 1996
   Ostium secundum ASD
   Wolff-Parkinson-White
   LBBB
   Dissecting aortic aneurysm

February 1996
Prolonged QT syndrome
Massive pulmonary embolism
Constrictive pericarditis
Cannon waves

October 1995
Pulmonary embolism and the pill
Mitral stenosis
Constrictive pericarditis
Wolff-Parkinson-White syndrome
Cardiac effects of alcohol abuse

July 1995
Cardiac complications of alcohol
Wolff-Parkinson-White syndrome
Ostium secundum ASD
Antibiotic prophylaxis of valves

February 1995
Diastolic dysfunction of LV
Fallot's tetralogy
Extension of an MI
Broad complex tachycardia

October 1994
Fixed splitting of the 2nd heart sound
Cyanotic heart disease
Ventricular tachycardia
Pulmonary embolus
Cardiac lesions causing reduced lung markings on
  chest X-ray

July 1994
    Causes of giant 'a' waves in the JVP
    Streptokinase therapy following myocardial
        infarction
    Conversion of atrial fibrillation to sinus rhythm
    Causes of reversed splitting of the second heart
        sound
    Acute myocardial infarction in the elderly

February 1994
    Causes of a dilated cardiomyopathy
    Causes of a right/left shunt
    Dissection of the aorta
    Cardiac tamponade

October 1993
    Mitral valve prolapse
    Pulmonary hypertension
    Cardiac valve lesions
    Loud first heart sound
    Features resulting from myocardial infarction

July 1993
    Uncontrolled atrial fibrillation
    Acute pericardial effusion
    Mitral stenosis
    Features of patent ductus arteriosus

February 1993
    Drugs causing torsades des pointes
    Aetiology of congestive cardiomyopathy
    Acute myocardial infarction
    Left bundle branch block
    Mitral stenosis
    Constrictive pericarditis

October 1992
Prolonged QT syndrome
Unstable angina
Aortic dissection
Cannon 'a' waves in the JVP

July 1992
Wolff-Parkinson-White syndrome
Left ventricular failure
Primary pulmonary hypertension
Constrictive pericarditis

February 1992
Recurrent pulmonary thromboembolism
Ventricular tachycardia
Early diastolic murmur
Giant 'a' waves in the JVP

October 1991
Constrictive pericarditis
Cardiovascular complications of alcohol
Hypertrophic cardiomyopathy

February 1991
Cardiac catheterization data
Infective endocarditis
The coronary circulation
Constrictive pericarditis
Wolff-Parkinson-White syndrome

Average 4–5 questions per exam. Numbers in brackets indicate the relative frequency of topics.

Valvular heart disease
- ❑ Heart sounds (4)
- ❑ Mitral stenosis (3)
- ❑ Valve lesions/murmurs (3)
- ❑ Antibiotic prophylaxis
- ❑ Catheterization data
- ❑ Mitral valve prolapse

Arrhythmias
- ❑ Wolff-Parkinson-White/SVT (6)
- ❑ Atrial fibrillation (3)
- ❑ Ventricular tachycardia (3)
- ❑ LBBB (2)
- ❑ Prolonged Q-T (2)
- ❑ Torsades des pointes

Pericardial disease
- ❑ Constrictive pericarditis (7)
- ❑ Cardiac tamponade (1)
- ❑ Pericardial effusion

IHD/heart muscle disease
- ❑ Myocardial infarction (6)
- ❑ Cardiomyopathy (4)
- ❑ Left ventricular failure (2)
- ❑ Unstable angina (2)
- ❑ Coronary bypass surgery
- ❑ Left ventricular hypertrophy
- ❑ Signs underlying heart disease

Congenital heart disease
❑ Cyanotic heart disease/Eisenmenger's (4)
❑ ASD (3)
❑ Patent ductus arteriosus
❑ VSD

Large vessel disease
❑ Pulmonary embolus (4)
❑ Aortic dissection (3)
❑ Pulmonary hypertension (3)

Miscellaneous
❑ Cannon 'a' waves in JVP (4)
❑ Alcohol and the heart (3)
❑ Carotid body/cardiac sympathetics (2)
❑ Coronary circulation
❑ Left atrial myxoma

October 1997
Erythema nodosum

July 1997
Pruritus

October 1996
Causes of purpura

July 1996
Erythema multiforme

February 1996
Associations with psoriasis

October 1995
Itchy papular rash

February 1995
Causes of pruritus

October 1994
Causes of photosensitivity

July 1993
Features of psoriasis

February 1993
Causes of skin lesions in the limbs

October 1992
Causes of perforating foot ulcers
Alopecia areata

July 1992
Skin manifestations of systemic disease
Photosensitive skin lesions

October 1991
Severe pruritus

February 1991
Erythema multiforme

DERMATOLOGY: REVISION CHECKLIST

Average only 1 question each or every other exam.
Numbers in brackets indicate the relative frequency of
topics.

Specific skin lesions
❏ Erythema multiforme (2)
❏ Psoriasis (2)
❏ Alopecia areata
❏ Erythema nodosum
❏ Papular rash
❏ Purpura

Systemic manifestations
❏ Pruritus (3)
❏ Photosensitivity (2)
❏ Skin manifestations of systemic disease

Miscellaneous
❏ Foot ulcers
❏ Lesions on limbs

October 1997
Glycosylated haemoglobin (HbA_1C) levels
Normal hormonal physiology
Raised T4 and TSH
IDDM
Serum markers in malignancy
Associations with short stature
SIADH

July 1997
Acromegaly
Polycystic ovary syndrome
Thyroid function tests
Diabetes mellitus
Prader-Willi syndrome

Jan 1997
Addison's disease
Thyroid carcinoma
IDDM
Hyperparathyroidism
Congenital adrenal hyperplasia
Ectopic ACTH/Cushing's syndrome

October 1996
Acromegaly
Diabetes mellitus
Hot thyroid nodule
Clinical associations of endocrine disease

July 1996
Cushing's syndrome
Addison's disease
Polycystic ovary syndrome
Endocrine changes of anorexia

February 1996
    Calcitonin
    Congenital adrenal hyperplasia
    Chromophobe adenoma
    Hypoglycaemia in diabetes
    SIADH
    Infertility and amenorrhoea

October 1995
    Elevated free thyroxine level
    Acromegaly
    Cushing's syndrome
    The insulin resistance syndrome

July 1995
    Graves' disease
    Acromegaly
    Raised parathyroid hormone

February 1995
    Hirsutism and amenorrhoea
    Vitamin D metabolism
    Hypothyroidism
    IDDM

October 1994
    Type II diabetes
    Addison's disease
    Parathyroid hormone-related protein
    Cushing's syndrome

Endocrinology

July 1994
Metabolism of thyroid hormone, T3
Microalbuminuria in diabetes
Cushing's syndrome
Associations of hyperprolactinaemia
Features of primary adrenal insufficiency

February 1994
Causes of hypoglycaemia
Causes of low free T4 levels
Acromegaly
Cushing's syndrome
Drugs which inhibit hepatic gluconeogenesis

October 1993
Hormones secreted by pituitary
Polycystic ovarian syndrome
Type I diabetes
Unilateral exophthalmos
Causes of abnormal ACTH release
Weight gain

July 1993
Features of insulin-induced hypoglycaemia
Polycystic ovary syndrome
Causes of excess sweating
Hypopituitarism

February 1993
Congenital adrenal hyperplasia
Papillary carcinoma of the thyroid
Physiological responses to hypoglycaemia

14

October 1992
    Cushing's syndrome
    Primary hyperparathyroidism

July 1992
    Short stature
    Calcitonin
    Insulinoma
    Hyperprolactinaemia
    Congenital adrenal hyperplasia

February 1992
    Inappropriate ADH secretion
    Myxoedema
    Chromophobe adenomas
    Low thyroxine levels

October 1991
    Insulin-dependent diabetes
    Serum thyroxine levels

February 1991
    Cushing's syndrome
    Thyroxine metabolism

Average 4 questions per exam. Numbers in brackets indicate the relative frequency of topics. (See also insulin, aldosterone secretion and ADH in *Basic Science* section.)

Diabetes and glycaemic control
❑ Diabetes (11)
❑ Hypoglycaemia (4)
❑ Glycosylated haemoglobin
❑ Hepatic gluconeogenesis
❑ Insulinoma

Adrenal disease
❑ Cushing's syndrome (8)
❑ Addison's disease (4)
❑ Congenital adrenal hyperplasia (4)
❑ ACTH action

Thyroid disease
❑ Thyroxine action/metabolism/TFTs (6)
❑ Thyroid cancer/nodule (3)
❑ Graves' disease/exophthalmos (2)
❑ Hypothyroidism (2)

Parathyroid disease
❑ PTH/hyperparathyroidism (4)
❑ Calcitonin (2)

Pituitary disease
❑ Acromegaly (5)
❑ Chromophobe adenoma (2)
❑ Hyperprolactinaemia (2)
❑ Hypopituitarism
❑ Pituitary hormones

Miscellaneous

- ❏ Polycystic ovary syndrome/infertility (4)
- ❏ SIADH (3)
- ❏ Short stature (2)
- ❏ Weight gain/Prader-Willi syndrome (2)
- ❏ Endocrine changes in anorexia
- ❏ Hirsutism
- ❏ Hormone physiology (including pregnancy)
- ❏ Sweating

October 1997
Portal vein thrombosis
Malignancy in ulcerative colitis
Crohn's disease
Coeliac disease
Protein-losing enteropathy
Reflux oesophagitis

July 1997
Intestinal absorption
Recurrent abdominal pain
Crohn's disease
Ulcerative colitis and colonic carcinoma
Hepatitis B

Jan 1997
Crohn's disease
Irritable bowel syndrome
Oesophageal reflux
Coeliac disease
Pancreatitis

October 1996
Intrahepatic cholestasis
Alcohol and the liver
Upper GI haemorrhage

July 1996
Protein-losing enteropathy
Acute pancreatitis
Primary biliary cirrhosis
Chronic liver disease

February 1996
Faecal occult blood detection
Gastric acid secretion
Urinary urobilinogen
Causes of diarrhoea
Viral hepatitis
Fulminant hepatic failure
Inflammatory bowel disease

October 1995
Gastrointestinal hormones
Acute gastrointestinal haemorrhage
Features of Whipple's disease

July 1995
Gilbert's syndrome
Achalasia
Associations of dysphagia
Primary biliary cirrhosis
Painful scrotal swelling

February 1995
Cellular effects of cholera toxin
Crohn's disease
Causes of villous atrophy
Oesophageal chest pain

October 1994
Gluten-sensitive enteropathy
Associations of oesophageal tumour
Crohn's disease
Features of the gastric proton pump
Carcinoid syndrome

July 1994
Ulcerative colitis
Acute pancreatitis
Pseudomembranous colitis
Carcinoma of the stomach

February 1994
Coeliac disease
Achalasia of the cardia
Primary biliary cirrhosis

October 1993
Irritable bowel syndrome
Gastrointestinal bleeding
Inflammatory bowel disease
Causes of acute pancreatitis

July 1993
Associations of ulcerative colitis
Associations of untreated coeliac disease
Investigations of oesophageal disease
Primary biliary cirrhosis

February 1993
Irritable bowel syndrome
Acute gastroenteritis
Crohn's disease
Subphrenic abscess
Coeliac disease
Causes of conjugated hyperbilirubinaemia

October 1992
Unconjugated hyperbilirubinaemia
Achalasia of the cardia
Uses of plain abdominal X-rays
Ulcerative colitis
Malabsorption syndrome

July 1992
Chronic liver disease
Bacterial colonization of the jejunum
Gastro-oesophageal reflux
Inflammatory bowel disease

February 1992
Causes of hepatic mass
Persistent vomiting
Cirrhosis of the liver
Malabsorption
Ulcerative colitis

February 1991
Acute pancreatitis
Gilbert's syndrome
Traveller's diarrhoea

Average 4 questions per exam. Numbers in brackets indicate the relative frequency of topics.

Liver disease
- ❑ Chronic liver disease (4)
- ❑ Jaundice (4)
- ❑ Primary biliary cirrhosis (4)
- ❑ Gilbert's syndrome (2)
- ❑ Hepatic mass/sub-phrenic abscess (2)
- ❑ Alcohol & liver
- ❑ Portal vein thrombosis

Small bowel disease/Malabsorption
- ❑ Coeliac disease (7)
- ❑ Malabsorption/protein-losing enteropathy (4)
- ❑ Cholera toxin/gastroenteritis (3)
- ❑ Carcinoid syndrome
- ❑ Whipple's disease
  (see also 'Crohn's disease' below)

Large bowel disorders
- ❑ Crohn's disease (6)
- ❑ Ulcerative colitis/colonic carcinoma (6)
- ❑ Irritable bowel syndrome (3)
- ❑ Diarrhoea (2)
- ❑ Inflammatory bowel disease - general (2)
- ❑ Pseudomembranous colitis

Oesophageal disease
- ❑ Gastro-oesophageal reflux/tests (4)
- ❑ Achalasia (3)
- ❑ Dysphagia/oesophageal tumour (2)
- ❑ Oesophageal chest pain

Stomach and pancreas
❑ Acute pancreatitis (5)
❑ Gastric acid secretion (2)
❑ Persistent vomiting
❑ Stomach cancer

Miscellaneous
❑ GI tract bleeding (4)
❑ Abdominal X-ray
❑ GI hormones
❑ Physiology of absorption
❑ Recurrent abdominal pain

October 1997
Abnormal karyotype
Chorionic villous sampling

July 1997
X-linked recessive inheritance
Autosomal dominant

Jan 1997
Abnormal karyotype (trinucleotide gene defects)
Down's syndrome
Turner's syndrome

October 1996
Abnormal karyotype (Turner's/Klinefelter's)
Inheritance pattern of various diseases

July 1996
Sex-linked recessive

February 1996
X-linked dominant conditions
Klinefelter's syndrome

October 1995
Klinefelter's syndrome

July 1995
Chromosomal defects
Turner's syndrome

February 1995
Genetic anticipation

October 1994
Klinefelter's syndrome

February 1994
Autosomal recessive inheritance

February 1993
Diseases associated with abnormal karyotype

October 1992
X-linked recessive conditions

July 1992
Down's syndrome

February 1992
Klinefelter's syndrome

October 1991
Turner's syndrome
Autosomal recessive conditions

February 1991
Abnormal karyotype

Average 2 questions every exam. Numbers in brackets indicate the relative frequency of topics.

Syndromes
- ❑ Klinefelter's syndrome (4)
- ❑ Turner's syndrome (3)
- ❑ Down's syndrome (2)

Modes of inheritance
- ❑ X-linked conditions (4)
- ❑ Autosomal recessive (2)
- ❑ Autosomal dominant
- ❑ Genetic anticipation
- ❑ Inheritance patterns (various)

Miscellaneous
- ❑ Abnormal karyotype (4)
- ❑ Chorionic villous sampling
- ❑ Chromosomal defects

October 1997
Post-splenectomy
Neutropaenia
Auto-immune thrombocytopaenia
Coombs +ve haemolysis
Prognosis of leukaemia/lymphoma
Vitamin B12 metabolism

July 1997
Sickle cell disease
Haemolytic anaemia
Macrocytosis with normoblastic erythropoiesis
Aplastic anaemia

Jan 1997
Haem synthesis
Polycythaemia
Erythropoiesis
Hereditary spherocytosis
Haemoglobin/oxygen

October 1996
Sickle cell syndrome
Paroxysmal nocturnal haemoglobinuria
CLL
Pernicious anaemia

July 1996
G-6-PD deficiency
Paroxysmal nocturnal haemoglobinuria
ALL
Thalassaemia

February 1996
Reticulocytosis
Haemolytic anaemia in an African
Prolonged bleeding time
Iron therapy for microcytic anaemia

October 1995
Iron storage compounds
Causes of pancytopenia/splenomegaly
Causes of thrombocytosis
Causes of basophilia
Usefulness of bone marrow trephine
Drug causes of methaemoglobinaemia

July 1995
Causes of hyposplenism
Haemoglobinopathies
Folate deficiency
Uses of fresh frozen plasma infusion
Von Willebrand's disease

February 1995
Reduced red cell folate
Intravascular haemolysis
Sideroblastic anaemia

October 1994
Hodgkin's disease
Leukaemia
Haemophilia A
Causes of thrombocytopenia

July 1994
Sickle cell disease
Hereditary spherocytosis
Haemolytic anaemia
Haematological causes of splenic enlargement
Haematological causes of hyperuricaemia
Hodgkin's lymphoma

February 1994
Differentiation of Hodgkin's/non-Hodgkin's
    lymphoma
Sideroblastic anaemia
Sickle cell disease
Associations of haemolytic anaemia
Iron metabolism

October 1993
Abnormal haem biosynthesis
Haematological abnormalities after splenectomy
Hodgkin's disease
Auto-immune thrombocytopenia

July 1993
Polycythaemia rubra vera
Hereditary spherocytosis
Prognosis in haematological diseases
Causes of neutropenia

February 1993
Investigation of anaemia
Thalassaemia major
Hodgkin's disease
Pancytopenia and splenomegaly

October 1992
ABO blood transfusion incompatibility
Anaemia and splenomegaly
Thrombocytosis
Haemolytic anaemia

July 1992
Acute lymphoblastic leukaemia
Haemophilia A
Bone infarction in haematological disease
Basophilia
Causes of a high reticulocyte count

February 1992
Haemolytic-uraemic syndrome
Causes of macrocytosis
Iron deficiency anaemia
Methaemoglobinaemia

October 1991
Folate deficiency
Pancytopenia
Iron treatment

February 1991
Red cell fragmentation
Pernicious anaemia
Eosinophilia
Complications of splenectomy

Average 4 questions per exam. Numbers in brackets indicate the relative frequency of topics.

Red cell physiology and anaemias
❑ Iron deficiency/metabolism/therapy (4)
❑ Macrocytosis/pernicious anaemia (4)
❑ Folate deficiency (3)
❑ Basophilia (2)
❑ Erythropoiesis/Hb physiology (2)
❑ Haem biosynthesis (2)
❑ Sideroblastic anaemia (2)
❑ Aplastic anaemia
❑ Investigation of anaemia
❑ Vitamin B12 metabolism

Haemolytic anaemia
❑ Haemolytic anaemia (7)
❑ Sickle cell/Haemoglobinopathy (7)
❑ Hereditary spherocytosis (2)
❑ Reticulocytosis (2)
❑ G-6-PD deficiency
❑ Haemolytic-uraemic syndrome
❑ Intravascular haemolysis

Bleeding disorders
❑ Thrombocytopaenia (3)
❑ Haemophilia (2)
❑ Bleeding time
❑ Fresh frozen plasma
❑ Von Willebrand's disease

Haematological malignancy
- ☐ Hodgkin's/Non-Hodgkin's lymphoma (5)
- ☐ Leukaemia (5)
- ☐ Pancytopaenia/splenomegaly (5)
- ☐ Polycythaemia (2)

Miscellaneous
- ☐ Hyposplenism (2)
- ☐ Methaemoglobinaemia (2)
- ☐ Neutropaenia (2)
- ☐ Thrombocytosis (2)
- ☐ Bone infarction
- ☐ Bone marrow test
- ☐ Eosinophilia
- ☐ Hyperuricaemia and haematological disease (see also *Metabolic Disease*)
- ☐ Paroxysmal nocturnal haemoglobinuria

October 1997
Type IV hypersensitivity
Mast cells

July 1997
CD4 lymphocytes
Polymerase chain reaction

Jan 1997
TNF

October 1996
T lymphocytes
Inflammatory mediators
Primary hypogammaglobulinaemia

July 1996
Complement
Immunoglobulin structure

February 1996
T cell deficiency
Pathogenic role of complement

October 1995
Tissue receptor antibodies and disease
Autoimmune disease
Tumour necrosis factor

July 1995
Gamma interferon
IgE and associated disease
Immunology of transplant rejection

February 1995
ANCA
Monoclonal gammopathy
Septicaemia after splenectomy

October 1994
T lymphocytes

July 1994
Interferon
IgA
Leucotrienes
Circulating immune complexes

February 1994
Hereditary angioneurotic oedema
Tumour necrosis factor
Monoclonal antibodies

October 1993
Inflammatory allergic reactions

July 1993
Angio-neurotic oedema
Deficiencies in cell-mediated immunity

October 1992
T lymphocytes
Type III hypersensitivity reactions

July 1992
Causes of low serum IgG
Specific tissue receptor antibodies

October 1991
    Causes of a low CH_{50}
    Primary hypogammaglobulinaemia

February 1991
    Precipitating antibodies in diagnosis

Coverage of immunology in the exam is increasing, with an average 2–3 questions per exam during the last 3 years. Numbers in brackets indicate the relative frequency of topics.

Cytokines
❑ Tumour necrosis factor (3)
❑ Interferon (2)
❑ Inflammatory mediators (general)
❑ Leukotrienes

Cellular immunity
❑ T lymphocytes/deficiency (5)
❑ Cell-mediated immunity (2)

Immunoglobulins/autoimmunity
❑ IgA/IgE/IgG (4)
❑ Autoimmune disease/ANCA (2)
❑ Hypogammaglobulinaemia (2)
❑ Monoclonal gammopathy (2)
❑ Tissue receptor antibodies (2)
❑ Circulating immune complexes
❑ Precipitating antibodies in diagnosis

Miscellaneous
❑ Complement/CH_{50} (3)
❑ Angioneurotic oedema (2)
❑ Hypersensitivity reactions (2)
❑ Mast cells
❑ Polymerase chain reaction
❑ Post-splenectomy
❑ Transplant rejection

October 1997
Faecal-oral transmission
Hepatitis A
Gonorrhoea
Insect vectors

July 1997
Insect vectors
Falciparum malaria
Bacteroides
Tetanus
Haemophilus influenza B

Jan 1997
HIV
EBV
Meningitis/CSF
NSU
Tetanus
Giardiasis

October 1996
Gonorrhoea
Hepatitis B
Falciparum malaria
Chickenpox
Salmonella typhi
Clinical presentation of different disease

July 1996
Infectious mononucleosis
Mumps
Toxoplasmosis
Cholera
Anaemia and chronic infection

February 1996
Adenovirus infection
Pneumonia
Malaria
Rubella
Chlamydia trachomatis

October 1995
Features of staphylococcal toxins
Infectious mononucleosis
Brucellosis
Infections causing diarrhoea
Toxoplasmosis

July 1995
Malaria
Parvovirus B19
Genital herpes

February 1995
Non-gonococcal urethritis
Chickenpox
Tuberculosis
Malaria
Hepatitis E

October 1994
Acute hepatitis B
Pneumocystis carinii
Malaria
Tetanus

July 1994
Infectious mononucleosis
Infections that cause eosinophilia
Giardia lamblia infection
Falciparum malaria
Brucellosis/Toxoplasmosis

February 1994
Hepatitis C
Features of rubella
Helicobacter pylori
Human prion disease
Chronic brucellosis

October 1993
Associations of HIV infection
Tropical fever and splenomegaly
Non-gonococcal urethritis
BCG immunization

July 1993
Lyme disease
Toxoplasmosis
Mumps
Infection with *Neisseria gonorrhoea*
Infectious mononucleosis
Causes of infectious disease in AIDS patients

February 1993
Cholera
Tetanus
Syphilis

October 1992
Brucellosis
Shistosomiasis
Measles encephalitis
AIDS

July 1992
Causes of rash, lymphadenopathy and fever
Infectious diarrhoea
Tuberculosis
Plasmodium malariae

February 1992
Rubella
Falciparum malaria

October 1991
Tuberculosis
Typhoid
Faecal oral transmission
Giardiasis
Chlamydia trachomatis
Hepatitis B infection

February 1991
Infectious mononucleosis
Transmission by insect bite

Average 4 questions per exam. Numbers in brackets indicate the relative frequency of topics.

Viral Infections
- ❏ Hepatitis (6)
- ❏ Infectious mononucleosis (6)
- ❏ Chickenpox/measles/mumps (5)
- ❏ AIDS/HIV (4)
- ❏ Adenovirus
- ❏ Genital herpes
- ❏ Parvovirus

Bacterial Infections
- ❏ Venereal disease (8)
- ❏ Brucellosis (4)
- ❏ TB/BCG (4)
- ❏ Tetanus (4)
- ❏ Toxoplasmosis (4)
- ❏ Typhoid/cholera (4)
- ❏ *Bacteroides*
- ❏ *Haemophilus influenza*
- ❏ *Helicobacter pylori*
- ❏ Lyme disease
- ❏ Meningitis
- ❏ Pneumonia
- ❏ Staphylococcus

Routes of infection
- ❏ Transmission by insect bite (3)
- ❏ Faecal-oral transmission (2)

Tropical and protozoal infections
- ❑ Malaria (9)
- ❑ Tropical fever/splenomegaly (2)
- ❑ Giardiasis
- ❑ *Pneumocystis carinii*
- ❑ Schistosomiasis

Miscellaneous
- ❑ *Chlamydia trachomatis* (2)
- ❑ Other infections/diarrhoea (2)
- ❑ Chronic infection and anaemia
- ❑ Infections and eosinophilia
- ❑ Prion disease

October 1997
Poisoning and metabolic acidosis

July 1997
Paracetamol overdose
Marfan's syndrome
Vitamin D metabolism
Hypernatraemia

Jan 1997
Osteoporosis
Elevated PSA
Poisoning

October 1996
Calcium homeostasis
Tricyclic poisoning

July 1996
Conjugated hyperbilirubinaemia
Metabolic alkalosis
Vitamin D metabolism
Theophylline poisoning

February 1996
Carbon monoxide poisoning
Excessive alcohol intake

October 1995
Causes of hypomagnesaemia
Malignant-neuroleptic syndrome
Wilson's disease

July 1995
Salicylate poisoning
Hypokalaemic acidosis
Homocystinuria
Causes of hyponatraemia

February 1995
Persistent vomiting
Hypomagnesaemia
Paget's disease
Tricyclic overdose
Hypophosphataemia
Vitamin D metabolism

October 1994
Overdose of paracetamol

July 1994
Metabolism of vitamin D
Iron toxicity
Chloride depletion
Hypothermia

February 1994
Causes of hypercalcaemia

October 1993
Raised alkaline phosphatase
Acute poisoning

July 1993
Features of theophylline overdose
Hypokalaemic acidosis
Kwashiorkor
Causes of hyperuricaemia

February 1993
   Achondroplasia
   Hypophosphataemic rickets
   Causes of hypokalaemia
   Osteoporosis

October 1992
   Osteoporosis
   Hypercarotinaemia

July 1992
   Causes of hypomagnesaemia
   Accidental hypothermia
   Paracetamol poisoning

February 1992
   Effects of heavy alcohol intake
   Osteoporosis
   Familial hypercholesterolaemia
   Causes of alkalosis
   Obesity
   Overdose of drugs

October 1991
   Polydypsia
   Wilson's disease

February 1991
   Familial hypercholesterolaemia
   $Alpha_1$-antitrypsin deficiency
   Hyperkalaemic acidosis
   Thiamine deficiency

Average 3 questions per exam. Numbers in brackets indicate the relative frequency of topics.

Overdose and poisoning
- ❑ Carbon monoxide/other poisoning (5)
- ❑ Salicylate/paracetamol overdose (4)
- ❑ Tricyclic/theophylline overdose (4)
- ❑ Excess alcohol (2)
- ❑ Iron toxicity

Disorders of bone
- ❑ Osteoporosis (4)
- ❑ Vitamin D metabolism (4)
- ❑ Achondroplasia
- ❑ Calcium homeostasis
- ❑ Increased alkaline phosphatase
- ❑ Increased prostate-specific antigen
- ❑ Paget's disease

Disorders of acid/base and electrolytes
- ❑ Hyper/hypokalaemia (4)
- ❑ Alkalosis/vomiting (3)
- ❑ Hypomagnesaemia (3)
- ❑ Hyponatraemia/chloride depletion (2)
- ❑ Hypophosphataemia (2)
- ❑ Hypercalcaemia
- ❑ Hypernatraemia
- ❑ Polydipsia

Inherited metabolic disorders
- ❑ Hypercholesterolaemia (2)
- ❑ Wilson's disease (2)
- ❑ Alpha$_1$-antitrypsin deficiency *(see also Basic Science)*
- ❑ Homocystinuria
- ❑ Malignant neuroleptic syndrome

Miscellaneous
- ❏ Hypothermia (2)
- ❏ Hypercarotenaemia
- ❏ Hyperuricaemia
- ❏ Kwashiorkor
- ❏ Marfan's syndrome
- ❏ Obesity
- ❏ Thiamine deficiency

October 1997
Polycystic kidney disease
Minimal change disease
Proximal RTA
Immune complex nephritis
Renal calculi
Serum creatinine

July 1997
Tubular physiology
Nephrotic syndrome
Retroperitoneal fibrosis

Jan 1997
Distal RTA
Contrast nephropathy
Nephrotic syndrome

October 1996
Renal physiology
Pre-renal uraemia
Acute glomerulonephritis
Steroid treatment of renal disease
Causes of renal medullary hypoxia

July 1996
Polycystic kidney disease
Anaemia of ESRF
Papillary necrosis
Diabetic nephropathy
Tubular sodium reabsorption

February 1996
Normal renal tubular function
Polycystic kidney disease
Hypocomplementaemia and glomerulonephritis
Minimal change disease

October 1995
Distal renal tubular acidosis
Renal vein thrombosis
Membranous nephropathy
Microalbuminuria in diabetes

July 1995
ARF and rhabdomyolysis
Macroscopic haematuria
Renal papillary necrosis

February 1995
Acute or chronic renal failure
Polycystic kidney disease
Nephrotic syndrome
Membranous glomerulonephritis

October 1994
Distal renal tubular acidosis
Nephrotic syndrome
Differentiation of acute and chronic renal failure
Hypertension and chronic renal failure

July 1994
Minimal change nephropathy
Factors affecting urine concentration
Chronic renal failure
Analgesic nephropathy

February 1994
Acute renal failure resulting from overdose
Adult polycystic kidney disease
Aetiology of chronic renal failure
Nephrotic range proteinuria
Uraemic osteodystrophy
Physiology of the proximal renal tubule

October 1993
Nephrotic syndrome
Diabetic microalbuminuria
Renal vein thrombosis
Normal renal tubular physiology

July 1993
Distal renal tubular acidosis
Nephrotic syndrome

February 1993
Renal water excretion
Haemolytic-uraemic syndrome

October 1992
Discolouration of the urine
Causes of nocturia
Lupus nephritis
Minimal change nephrotic syndrome

July 1992
Renal papillary necrosis
Nephrotic range proteinuria
Causes of acute on chronic renal failure

February 1992
Causes of polyuria
Membranous glomerulonephritis

October 1991
Acute renal failure and rhabdomyolysis
Nephrotic syndrome

February 1991
Macroscopic haematuria
Papillary necrosis
Membranous glomerulonephritis
Haemolytic uraemic syndrome
Drugs in renal failure

Average 3–4 questions per exam. Numbers in brackets indicate the relative frequency of topics.

Nephrotic syndrome/related glomerulonephritis
❑ Nephrotic syndrome (9)
❑ Membranous glomerulonephritis (4)
❑ Minimal Change disease (4)
❑ Hypocomplementaemia & glomerulonephritis (2)
❑ Renal vein thrombosis (2)
❑ Acute glomerulonephritis
❑ SLE nephritis

Renal failure
❑ Acute renal failure (4)
❑ Acute versus chronic (3)
❑ Chronic renal failure (3)
❑ Haemolytic-uraemic syndrome (2)
❑ Rhabdomyolysis (2)
❑ Anaemia in renal failure
❑ Contrast nephropathy

Urinary abnormalities
❑ Macroscopic haematuria (2)
❑ Discolouration of the urine
❑ Nocturia
❑ Polyuria

Basic renal physiology
❑ Normal renal physiology/function (6)
❑ Water excretion/urinary concentration (2)
❑ Serum creatinine

Miscellaneous
- ❑ Distal renal tubular acidosis (5)
- ❑ Renal papillary necrosis (4)
- ❑ Diabetic nephropathy (3)
- ❑ Analgesic nephropathy
- ❑ Polycystic kidney disease
- ❑ Renal calculi
- ❑ Renal osteodystrophy
- ❑ Retroperitoneal fibrosis
- ❑ Steroid therapy in renal disease

October 1997
Sixth cranial nerve
Lesion of medial cord of brachial plexus
Amyotrophic lateral sclerosis
Hemiplegic stroke
Creutzfeldt-Jakob disease
Memory loss

July 1997
Transection of sciatic nerve
Facial nerve lesion
Multiple sclerosis or vitamin B12 deficiency
Chronic subdural haematoma
Essential tremor

Jan 1997
Herpes encephalitis
Benign intracranial hypertension
Cerebral infarction
Pupillary light reflex
Facial nerve

October 1996
Chronic subdural haematoma
Oligoclonal bands in CSF
Pseudoseizures
Migraine
Myasthenia gravis
Nerve root innervation of peripheral muscles
Posterior column fibres

July 1996
Multiple sclerosis
Facial weakness
Wernicke's encephalopathy
Midbrain syndrome (Parinaud's)
Risk factors for CVA

February 1996
Lesion of 7th cranial nerve
Posterior interosseous nerve
Temporal lobe epilepsy
Paraesthesia
Duchenne muscular dystrophy
Multiple sclerosis

October 1995
Median nerve lesion
Section of posterior nerve roots
Normal pressure hydrocephalus
Guillain-Barré syndrome
Parkinson's disease

July 1995
Pyramidal tracts
Down-beat nystagmus
Radial nerve in upper arm
Cerebral circulatory disorders
Encephalitis
Central pontine myelinolysis
Prognosis of head injury

February 1995
   Drug causes of dyskinesia
   Finger weakness
   Lesion of pre-frontal cortex
   Lumbar puncture
   Dementia
   Vertigo

October 1994
   Hemiplegic migraine
   Cerebral control of finger movements
   Causes of cerebral abscess
   CNS involvement in AIDS
   Complete third nerve palsy
   Causes of ataxia
   Autonomic neuropathy
   Features of cervical spondylosis

July 1994
   Features of a parietal lobe lesion
   Lesion of the sixth cranial nerve
   Anatomical pathways for the pupillary light reflex
   Duchenne muscular dystrophy
   Causes of truncal ataxia
   Causes of intracranial calcification

February 1994
   Internuclear ophthalmoplegia
   Prognostic indicators in multiple sclerosis
   Prognosis of head injury
   Dementia
   Features of myotonic dystrophy
   Neurological tracts within the spinal cord

October 1993

Duchenne muscular dystrophy
Superior oblique muscle palsy
Lateral medullary syndrome
Innervation of the muscles of the hand
Transient ischaemic attacks

July 1993

Lesion of the sciatic nerve
Causes of down-beat nystagmus
Neurological prognosis after head injury

February 1993

Causes of muscle fasciculation
Chronic subdural haematoma
Dystrophia myotonica
Lesion of the facial nerve
Cranial nerves carrying parasympathetic fibres
Benign intracranial hypertension
Occlusion of the posterior cerebral artery

October 1992

Section of the dorsal interosseus nerve
Pseudo-fits
Multiple sclerosis
Guillain-Barré syndrome
Bulbar palsy
Temporal lobe epilepsy

July 1992

Facial nerve lesion
Headache
Nerve root innervation of muscles
Cranial nerve lesions
Brain tumour

February 1992
    Duchenne muscular dystrophy
    Section of the posterior nerve roots
    Causes of nystagmus
    Migraine
    CSF lymphocytosis
    Alzheimer's disease
    Recent memory loss
    Seventh cranial nerve

October 1991
    Transection of the facial nerve
    Benign essential tremor
    Lesions of the posterior spinal ganglia

February 1991
    Dysarthria
    Alzheimer's disease
    Combined upper/lower motor neurone lesion
    Damage to the median nerve
    EEG abnormalities

Average 5–6 questions per exam, including anatomy of the nervous system (excluded from Basic Sciences section). Numbers in brackets indicate the relative frequency of topics.

Abnormalities of brain & cerebral circulation
- ❏ Dementia/Alzheimer's (5)
- ❏ Transient ischaemic attacks/stroke (4)
- ❏ Benign intracranial hypertension/brain tumour (3)
- ❏ Head injury (3)
- ❏ Lateral medullary/circulatory syndromes (3)
- ❏ Subdural haematoma (3)
- ❏ Encephalitis (2)
- ❏ Parietal lobe/frontal cortical lesion (2)
- ❏ Temporal lobe epilepsy (2)
- ❏ Amnesia
- ❏ Central pontine myelinolysis
- ❏ Cerebral abscess
- ❏ Creutzfeldt-Jakob disease
- ❏ EEG
- ❏ Intracranial calcification
- ❏ Midbrain (Parinaud's) syndrome
- ❏ Normal pressure hydrocephalus
- ❏ Wernicke's encephalopathy

Spinal cord and peripheral nerve anatomy & lesions
- ❏ Innervation of specific muscles (4)
- ❏ Median nerve/brachial plexus (3)
- ❏ Posterior nerve root/spinal ganglia lesions (3)
- ❏ Dorsal interosseous nerve (2)
- ❏ Guillain-Barré (2)
- ❏ Pyramidal tracts/posterior column pathways (2)
- ❏ Sciatic nerve lesion (2)
- ❏ Autonomic neuropathy
- ❏ Cervical spondylosis

❏ Motor neuron disease
❏ Paraesthesia
❏ Spinal cord lesions

Cranial nerve anatomy & lesions
❏ Facial nerve (6)
❏ Cranial nerve lesions (5)
❏ Third nerve palsy/pupillary reflex (3)
❏ Bulbar palsy
❏ Internuclear ophthalmoplegia
❏ 4th nerve palsy

Dyskinesias
❏ Ataxia (2)
❏ Benign essential tremor (2)
❏ Dyskinesia
❏ Parkinson's disease

Muscular disorders
❏ Duchenne muscular dystrophy (4)
❏ Myotonic dystrophy (2)
❏ Myaesthenia gravis

Miscellaneous
❏ Multiple sclerosis (5)
❏ Headache/migraine (4)
❏ Lumbar puncture/CSF (3)
❏ Nystagmus (3)
❏ Pseudofits (2)
❏ Vertigo/dysarthria (2)
❏ CNS involvement in AIDS

July 1996
Hemianopia

July 1995
Diabetic retinopathy

February 1995
Central retinal vein occlusion

October 1993
Background diabetic retinopathy

February 1993
Uveitis

October 1992
Causes of painful ophthalmoplegia

July 1992
Central scotoma

February 1992
Diabetic eye changes

October 1991
Cataracts

February 1991
Papilloedema

Average 1 question every 2 examinations. Numbers in brackets indicate the relative frequency of topics.

Retinal and optic disc disease
❑ Diabetic eye changes (3)
❑ Central retinal vein occlusion
❑ Papilloedema

Visual field defects
❑ Central scotoma
❑ Hemianopia

Miscellaneous
❑ Cataracts
❑ Painful ophthalmoplegia
❑ Uveitis

October 1997
Drugs causing bronchospasm
Lithium
Drugs and their respective side effects
Drug interactions with oral contraceptives
Verapamil
Drugs that cause or aggravate skin disorders

July 1997
Selective serotonin reuptake inhibitors
Griseofulvin
Acyclovir
Amiodarone
Oral hypoglycaemics

Jan 1997
Hepatic enzyme inducers
Drugs in pregnancy
Causes of haemolytic anaemia
Drug combinations
Metronidazole
Retinoids

October 1996
Drugs and breast-feeding
Drugs in pregnancy
ACE inhibitors
Drugs causing hypokalaemia
Tubular sites of diuretic action
Radio-iodine treatment
ß2 agonist actions

July 1996
Polymorphisms/drug metabolism
Gabapentin
Cimetidine
Lithium
Drugs and porphyria
Drugs causing hyperprolactinaemia

February 1996
Drugs in breast-feeding mothers
Drugs causing hypothyroidism
Adverse reactions from combination drugs
Adverse effects of thiazides

October 1995
Drugs which exacerbate asthma
Adverse effects of drugs
Drugs which interact with warfarin

July 1995
Contraindications for ACE inhibition
Mechanisms of drug action
Atenolol
Drugs and increase in digoxin level
HMG CoA-reductase inhibitors

February 1995
Amiodarone
Drug interactions
Azidothymidine (AZT)
Dosage reduction in renal failure

October 1994
Sumatriptan
Etidronate
Selective alpha$_1$ blockade

July 1994
  Sodium valproate
  Oral iron therapy
  Drugs enhancing the action of dopamine
  Toxic effects of amiodarone
  Side effects of thiazides

February 1994
  Sulphasalazine
  L-dopa
  Terminal care pain control with morphine
  Effects of lithium
  Gentamicin therapy
  Effects of anti-convulsants
  Drugs requiring dosage reduction in renal failure
  Radio-iodine treatment

October 1993
  Interactions between drugs and the contraceptive
    pill
  Drugs and adverse effects
  ACE inhibitors
  Non-steroidal anti-inflammatory agents
  Side effects of sulphasalazine

July 1993
  Enzyme inducers
  Side effects of isoretinoin
  Penicillamine
  Metronidazole

February 1993
  Cimetidine
  Digoxin overdose
  Drugs and acute intermittent porphyria

October 1992
Enalapril
Hypokalaemic side effects of drug therapy
Serious drug interactions
Drug induced hypothyroidism

July 1992
Griseofulvin
Mechanisms of antibiotic action
Chlorpromazine
Amitriptyline

February 1992
Drugs causing gynaecomastia
Hazardous drug combinations
Cisplatin side effects
Drugs crossing the placenta
Oral hypoglycaemics

October 1991
Interactions with warfarin
Unwanted effects of digoxin
Thiazide diuretics
Unwanted effects of drugs
Drugs causing convulsions

February 1991
Amiodarone
Carbimazole
Drugs in pregnancy
Drugs interacting with prolactin secretion
Oral contraceptive pill side effects

Average 4–5 questions per exam. Numbers in brackets indicate the relative frequency of topics.

Interactions/dose adjustment
☐ Drug interactions (10)
☐ Pregnancy/breast-feeding (7)
☐ Adverse effects – general (4)
☐ Dose adjustment in renal failure (3)
☐ Drugs in porphyria
☐ Polymorphism of drug metabolism

Specific side effects of drugs
☐ Asthma exacerbation (2)
☐ Causing hypothyroidism (2)
☐ Gynaecomastia/hyperprolactinaemia (2)
☐ Hepatic enzyme inducers (2)
☐ Hypokalaemia (2)
☐ Aggravation of skin disorders
☐ Convulsions
☐ Haemolytic anaemia

Fundamental pharmacology
☐ Mechanisms of drug/antibiotic action (2)

Most frequently considered individual agents
☐ Antipsychotics/depressants (5)
☐ ACE inhibitors (4)
☐ Amiodarone (4)
☐ Thiazides (4)
☐ Anti-convulsants (3)
☐ Digoxin (3)
☐ Lithium (3)
☐ Sulphasalazine (2)
☐ Metronidazole
☐ Radio-iodine

Pharmacology

Other 'topical' agents
- ❏ Azidothymidine (AZT)
- ❏ Cimetidine
- ❏ Gentamicin
- ❏ Griseofulvin
- ❏ HMG Co-A reductase inhibitor
- ❏ L-dopa
- ❏ Metronidazole
- ❏ Penicillamine
- ❏ Retinoic acid
- ❏ Warfarin

October 1997
Anxiety
Depression in the elderly
Psychiatric manifestations of organic disease
Manifestations of psychiatric disease in adolescents

July 1997
Acute confusional state
Mania
Schizophrenia

Jan 1997
Panic attack
Alcohol dependence
Eating disorders
Affective disorders

October 1996
Anorexia nervosa
Features of depressive illness
Differentiation of functional or organic disorder

July 1996
Psychiatric manifestations of organic disease
Obsessional neurosis
Schizophrenia
Endocrine causes of psychiatric disease

February 1996
Anorexia nervosa
Dementia/depression
Somatization syndrome
Schizophrenia

October 1995
Bulimia nervosa
Obsessional neurosis
Insomnia
Features of mania

July 1995
Anorexia nervosa
Depression in the elderly
Mania
Acute confusional state

February 1995
Depression
Schizophrenia
Anorexia nervosa
Narcolepsy

October 1994
Causes of visual hallucinations
Acute mania
Features of delirium tremens
Emotional lability

July 1994
Schizophrenia
Dementia
Neurosis
Psychogenic symptoms

February 1994
Risk of successful suicide
Features of obsessive-compulsive disorders
Features suggesting an organic basis for psychiatric
symptoms

October 1993
Adult alcohol dependency syndrome
Paranoid delusions
Neuropsychiatric symptoms and organic disease
Causes of sleep disturbance

July 1993
Acute schizophrenia
Obsessional neurosis
Depression/dementia
Bulimia

February 1993
Endogenous depression
Obsessive-compulsive state
Mania
Schizophrenia

October 1992
Anorexia nervosa
Narcolepsy

July 1992
Conversion syndromes
Disorders of affect
Persecutory delusions
Eating disorders

February 1992
Schizophrenia
Organic psychiatric symptoms

October 1991
Anorexia nervosa
Mania

February 1991
    Anxiety
    Depression in the elderly
    Anorexia nervosa

Average 4 questions per exam. Numbers in brackets indicate the relative frequency of topics.

Psychotic disorders
- ❏ Schizophrenia (8)
- ❏ Depression (7)
- ❏ Mania (6)
- ❏ Hallucinations/delusions (3)

Anxiety states/compulsive disorders
- ❏ Neurosis/psychogenic/conversion disorders (5)
- ❏ Obsessional/compulsive disorders (5)
- ❏ Panic attack

Eating disorders
- ❏ Anorexia nervosa (9)
- ❏ Bulimia (2)

Other cognitive disorders
- ❏ Differentiation of dementia and depression (3)
- ❏ Acute confusional state (2)

Miscellaneous
- ❏ Psychiatric manifestations of organic disease (6)
- ❏ Alcohol dependency (3)
- ❏ Insomnia (2)
- ❏ Narcolepsy (2)
- ❏ Endocrine causes of psychiatric disease
- ❏ Psychiatric manifestations in adolescence

October 1997
Sleep apnoea syndrome
Investigations prior to surgery for bronchial cancer
Mycoplasma pneumonia

July 1997
Lung function tests
Forced hyperventilation
Normal pulmonary physiology/anatomy
Cystic fibrosis
Farmer's lung

Jan 1997
Asthma
Extrinsic allergic alveolitis
Bronchiectasis
Pulmonary fibrosis

October 1996
Cystic fibrosis
Apical lung fibrosis
Sarcoidosis
Risks of bronchial carcinoma
Causes of lobar consolidation

July 1996
Asthma
Bronchiectasis
Pulmonary function tests
Carcinoma of bronchus/surgery

February 1996
    Sleep apnoea syndrome
    Pulmonary complications of SLE
    Pulmonary aspergillosis
    Pneumothorax

October 1995
    Bronchopulmonary aspergillosis
    Bronchial carcinoid tumour
    Extrinsic allergic alveolitis
    Mycoplasma pneumoniae

July 1995
    Adult respiratory distress syndrome
    Exercise-induced asthma
    Obstructive sleep apnoea

February 1995
    Community-acquired pneumonia
    Oat cell bronchial carcinoma
    Pulmonary eosinophilia

October 1994
    Type I respiratory failure
    Causes of calcification on chest X-ray
    Bullous emphysema
    Pulmonary manifestation of SLE

July 1994
    Transfer factor
    Lung perfusion scanning
    Indications for long-term oxygen therapy
    Community acquired pneumonia

February 1994
Causes of pulmonary cavitation
Emphysema
Small cell carcinoma of the lung

October 1993
Causes of respiratory failure
Sarcoidosis
Transfer factor
Causes of respiratory crackles on auscultation
Bronchiectasis

July 1993
Fibrosing alveolitis
Predisposition to bronchial carcinoma
Normal pulmonary physiology

February 1993
Pulmonary aspergillosis
Severe asthma attack
Causes of bronchiectasis

October 1992
Acute bronchiolitis
Adult respiratory distress syndrome
Lung function tests
Obstructive sleep apnoea
Occupational asthma
Physiological characteristics of normal ventilation

July 1992
Pancoast's tumour of lung
Asbestosis
Sarcoidosis
Abnormalities of chest X-ray

February 1992
 Respiratory distress syndrome
 Extrinsic allergic alveolitis
 Atypical pneumonias
 Surgery for lung cancer
 Aetiology of chronic respiratory disease

October 1991
 Mycoplasma pneumoniae
 Respiratory manifestations of rheumatoid arthritis
 Clubbing
 Type II respiratory failure
 Psittacosis
 Bronchial carcinoid syndrome
 Extrinsic allergic alveolitis

February 1991
 Viral respiratory infections
 Spontaneous pneumothorax
 Alveolar hyperventilation
 Farmer's lung
 Obstructive sleep apnoea

RESPIRATORY DISEASE: REVISION CHECKLIST

Average 4 questions per exam. Numbers in brackets indicate the relative frequency of topics.

Respiratory infections
- [ ] Pneumonia (7)
- [ ] Broncho-pulmonary aspergillosis (3)
- [ ] Acute bronchiolitis
- [ ] Psittacosis
- [ ] Viral infections

Lung cancer
- [ ] Bronchial carcinoma (5)
- [ ] Surgery for cancer (3)
- [ ] Pancoast's tumour
- [ ] Small cell cancer

Pulmonary physiology
- [ ] Lung function tests (4)
- [ ] Normal physiology (3)
- [ ] Transfer factor (2)
- [ ] Forced hyperventilation

End-stage lung disease
- [ ] Respiratory failure (4)
- [ ] Long-term oxygen

Interstitial lung disease/fibrosis
- [ ] Extrinsic allergic alveolitis (6)
- [ ] Bronchiectasis (4)
- [ ] ARDS (3)
- [ ] Sarcoidosis (3)
- [ ] Emphysema (2)
- [ ] Fibrosing alveolitis (2)
- [ ] Pulmonary fibrosis (2)
- [ ] Asbestosis
- [ ] Cystic fibrosis

Miscellaneous
- ❑ Asthma (5)
- ❑ Sleep-apnoea syndrome (5)
- ❑ Autoimmune disease and lung (3)
- ❑ Abnormal chest X-ray (2)
- ❑ Pneumothorax (2)
- ❑ Lung cavitation
- ❑ Pulmonary eosinophilia

October 1997
Osteoarthritis

July 1997
HLA B27 associated disease
Anti-phospholipid syndrome
Causes of arthropathy

Jan 1997
SLE
Rheumatoid arthritis

October 1996
Polymyalgia rheumatica

July 1996
Pseudogout
Arthralgia
Wegener's granulomatosis

February 1996
Polymyalgia rheumatica
Antiphospholipid syndrome

October 1995
SLE
Systemic sclerosis and the gut

July 1995
Behçet's disease
Hypertrophic osteoarthropathy

February 1995
Seropositive rheumatoid arthritis

October 1994
   Rheumatoid arthritis
   Vasculitic disease

July 1994
   Polymyalgia rheumatica
   Central nervous system abnormalities in SLE

February 1994
   Features of Reiter's syndrome
   Rheumatoid arthritis
   Polymyositis

October 1993
   SLE
   Associations with ankylosing spondylitis
   Neurological complications of rheumatoid arthritis
   Reiter's disease

July 1993
   Causes of peri-articular calcification
   SLE

February 1993
   Reiter's syndrome
   Cranial arteritis

October 1992
   Causes of arthralgia

July 1992
   SLE

February 1992
Causes of arthritis
Wegener's granulomatosis

October 1991
Behçet's disease

February 1991
Seropostive rheumatoid arthritis
Polymyalgia rheumatica
Digital gangrene

Average 2 questions per exam. Numbers in brackets indicate the relative frequency of topics.

Auto-immune disease
☐ Rheumatoid arthritis (7)
☐ SLE (7)
☐ Wegener's granulomatosis (2)

Other vasculitides
☐ Polymyalgia rheumatica (4)
☐ Cranial arteritis
☐ Vasculitic disease

Other arthritides
☐ Reiter's syndrome (3)
☐ Ankylosing spondylitis/HLA B27 (2)
☐ Arthralgia (2)
☐ Behçet's disease (2)
☐ Arthropathy (general)
☐ Hypertrophic osteo-arthropathy
☐ Osteoarthritis
☐ Pseudogout

Miscellaneous
☐ Anti-phospholipid syndrome (3)
☐ Digital gangrene
☐ Peri-articular calcification
☐ Systemic sclerosis

October 1997
Standard error and deviation

July 1997
Statistical errors (type I & II)

Jan 1997
Significance tests

October 1996
Specificity/sensitivity of clinical trials

July 1996
Tests of significance

February 1996
Normal distribution

October 1995
Standard deviation

February 1995
Significance tests

October 1994
Features of a normal distribution

July 1994
Statistical tests in a normal distribution

February 1994
Skewed distribution

October 1993
Specificity of clinical trials

July 1993
    Chi-squared test

February 1993
    Tests of significance

October 1992
    Standard deviation

February 1992
    Tests of significance

October 1991
    Significance tests

February 1991
    Normal distribution

STATISTICS: REVISION CHECKLIST

Average 1 question per exam. Numbers in brackets
indicate the relative frequency of topics.

Statistical populations
❑ Normal distribution (4)
❑ Standard deviation (3)
❑ Skewed distribution

Tests of significance
❑ Significance tests (6)
❑ Chi-square test
❑ Type I and II errors

Miscellaneous
❑ Specificity of clinical trials (2)

PASTEST: the key to exam success, the key to your future.
PasTest is dedicated to helping doctors to pass their professional examinations. We have 25 years of specialist experience in medical education and over 3000 doctors attend our revision courses each year.

Experienced lecturers:
Many of our lecturers are also examiners and teach in a lively and interesting way in order to:
✓ reflect current trends in exams
✓ give plenty of mock exam practice
✓ provide essential advice on exam technique

Outstanding accelerated learning:
Our up-to-date and relevant course material includes MCQs, colour slides, X-rays, ECGs, EEGs, clinical cases, data interpretations, mock exams, vivas and extensive course notes which provide:
✓ hundreds of high quality questions with detailed answers and explanations
✓ succinct notes, diagrams and charts

Personal attention:
Active participation is encouraged on these courses, so in order to give personal tuition and to answer individual questions our course numbers are limited. Book early to avoid disappointment.

Choice of courses:
PasTest has developed a wide range of high quality interactive courses in different cities around the UK to suit your individual needs.

What other students have said about our courses:
'Absolutely brilliant - I would not have passed without it! Thank you.'
Dr Charitha Rajapakse, London.
'Excellent, enjoyable, extremely hard work but worth every penny.'
Dr Helen Binns, Oxford.

For further details contact:
PasTest, Egerton Court, Parkgate Estate, Knutsford, Cheshire WA16 8DX, UK.

Telephone: 01565 755226   Fax: 01565 650264
e-mail: pastest@dial.pipex.com
web site: http:\\www.pastest.co.uk

PasTest are the leading independent specialists in post-graduate medical education. We publish a wide range of revision books including:

MCQs in Basic Medical Sciences for MRCP 1
> 300 exam-based MCQs with correct answers and detailed explanatory notes

MRCP 1 Practice Exams: 2nd edition
> Five complete MCQ Papers (300 MCQs) covering favourite Royal College topics

MRCP 1 MCQ Revision Book: 3rd edition
> 300 MCQs arranged by subject with correct answers and teaching notes, plus one complete mock exam

MRCP 1 MCQs with Key Topic Summaries: 2nd edition
> 200 exam-based MCQs with correct answers and 200 key topic summaries

Explanations to the RCP Past Papers
> Correct answers and teaching notes related to the Royal College Green and Blue books of actual past exam questions

MRCP Part 1 MCQ Pocket Books
> Each pocket-sized book contains 100 MCQs on favourite Membership topics

For full details of all our revision books contact PasTest today on **01565 755226** for a free copy of our current book catalogue and price list. Books sent by return of post worldwide.

ORDER FORM

Please send me:

- ❏ One copy of **MCQs in Basic Medical Sciences** £15.95
- ❏ One copy of **MCQ Practice Exams**: 2nd Edition £14.95
- ❏ One copy of **MCQ Revision Book**: 3rd Edition £14.95
- ❏ One copy of **MCQs with Key Topic Summaries**: 2nd Edition £14.95
- ❏ One copy of **Explanations to the Green Book** £12.00
- ❏ One copy of **Explanations to the Blue Book** £4.50 inc. P&P
- ❏ One copy of **Pocket Book 1: Cardiology, Resp. Med.** £7.50
- ❏ One copy of **Pocket Book 2: Neurology, Psychiatry** £7.50
- ❏ One copy of **Pocket Book 3: Gastro, Endo, Renal Med.** £7.50
- ❏ One copy of **Pocket Book 4: Rheum, Immun, Inf. Dis.** £7.50
- ❏ One copy of **Pocket Book 5: Basic Sciences** £7.50
- ❏ Order all **5 Pocket Books** for only: £35.00

Postage UK: £2.50 Europe: £3.50 Outside Europe: £7.00

Please add cost of postage:
UK: £1.30 for the first book plus 80p for each additional book
Europe: £2.00 for the first book plus 80p for each additional book
Outside Europe: £3.50 for the first book plus £2.30 for each additional book

Name: . . . .

Address: . . . .

. . . . .Daytime telephone no: . . . .

- ❏ I enclose a cheque/money order payable in pounds sterling to PasTest. (Please write your cheque guarantee card number and expiry date clearly on the back of the cheque.)
- ❏ Please debit my Access/Visa/Switch card

Card number . . . . .Signature. . . . .

Expiry date . . . . .Switch Issue Number . . . .

**PasTest, Egerton Court, Parkgate Estate,
Knutsford, Cheshire WA16 8DX, UK**
CREDIT CARD HOTLINE: 01565 755226
e-mail: pastest@dial.pipex.com
web site: http:\\www.pastest.co.uk